I0712049

THIN THINKING

No Diet Weight Loss

ROB SALTER

authorHOUSE®

AuthorHouse™ UK
1663 Liberty Drive
Bloomington, IN 47403 USA
www.authorhouse.co.uk
Phone: UK TFN: 0800 0148641 (Toll Free inside the UK)
*   UK Local: (02) 0369 56322 (+44 20 3695 6322 from outside the UK)*

Published by AuthorHouse 06/10/2024

ISBN: 979-8-8230-8810-7 (sc)
ISBN: 979-8-8230-8811-4 (e)

Library of Congress Control Number: 2024911620

Print information available on the last page.

Any people depicted in stock imagery provided by Getty Images are models, and such images are being used for illustrative purposes only. Certain stock imagery © Getty Images.

This book is printed on acid-free paper.

CONTENTS

INTRODUCTION

There are a number of approaches to natural weight loss, so what makes this one different?

For the sake of clarity, you can use self-hypnosis or you can eat mindfully or intuitively. When I began my own research into weight loss without the heart-breaking disappointment of failing on yet another diet, I also tried elements of these other systems and approaches and found that, to an extent, they did work … until they didn't of course.

The approach that I settled on however, owes more to a little known body of work called The Three Principles. This method is sometimes referred to as the 'inside out understanding of life', meaning that it is based on a understanding that as thinking beings, we create our own unique experience of life, moment by moment, via our thinking.

The Three Principles derives its power from a natural process of 'insight', that is to say an experience of yourself as a thinking being, often accompanied by a deep sense of relaxation and wellbeing.

I began to use this system at first to heal my relationships and to manage stress but over time I began to have insights about how my body worked and how my thinking around food was sabotaging my weight loss progress.

I share many of my insights in this book.

The power of this approach, in my view is that once you have seen something about your relationship towards food for example, you can't un-see it. Your insights are as unique as you are and they are equally powerful and life changing for everyone.

I have spoken to and listened to people who have come off drugs or turned their lives around after prison for example, all as a result of the profound impact of their individual insights.

Insights, generally are predicated upon a realisation that nothing outside of me can create permanent change and that —as a corollary-only change from the inside out can possibly last.

Personally, as a result of my own insights, I now know that:

- Diets are a misunderstanding – restricting a food group is an 'outside-in' approach

- Using exercise only to lose body fat is a misunderstanding – adding in one form of exercise

     ROB SALTER

or another in order to create permanent change is an 'outside-in' approach

- Comfort eating is a misunderstanding – using something external to you, to change your internal mood makes no sense.

This series of insights has set me against the vast majority of conventional wisdom promoted by the diet and exercise industry. My hope is that industry professionals will be far sighted enough to incorporate some of this wisdom into their current work.

My hope is also that the average reader will find in these pages, a spark of insight which will lead them to a clearer understanding of their own relationship to food and exercise and help them to naturally shed some of their excess weight.

However, you choose to use this book, please approach it with an open mind and heart and an expectation that your innate health will show you the way forwards.

THIS BOOK IN TEN SENTENCES

1. Most people's taste buds are an undiscovered country—
    get to know yours.

2. Slow down and count your chews—try getting to thirty.

3. Shop for food based on the tastes you like.

4. Your body has a perfect system for keeping you slim.
    You just haven't listened to it.

5. Your mind wants to feed you more than your body needs.

6. Any insight you have leads you to see that life is coming
    from and not *at* you.

7. Once you see that you create your reality via thought,
    you can't unsee it.

8. It's not about what but how you eat—don't restrict or
    worry about 'bad' food.

9. Your 'naturally' slim friends are your role models.

10. Fasting or fruit till noon and after dinner can speed up
    this process.

NO ONE TRANSFORMS ANYONE

I can't make you thin (but you can).

During the research for the initial programme that formed the basis of this book, I came across a really helpful book called *Mindfullness* by Elaine Hilides. This seemed to me to be the first attempt by a three-principles practitioner to write about weight loss. When she was focused on NLP and hypnosis as tools for change, Elaine had been an assistant at Paul McKenna's workshops, named after the book *I Can Make You Thin.*

She makes the observation that many people did lose weight as a result of this well-known workshop and many did not. Paul suggests very simple rules for weight loss, very much in line with the insights that I had about my own body having a perfect system for keeping me slim, if I only used it.

He would speak about only eating when you are hungry and stopping when you are full and eating consciously, or mindfully, as I would put it. As Elaine comments, these methods really are just common sense.

On reflection, I now see that people using Paul's methods may not have lost weight for the same reason that my early clients did not lose weight either. They were, on some unconscious level, relying on me to lose the weight for them (although none of them would acknowledge this, of course), and the insights that Paul was sharing were *his* insights as opposed to *theirs*.

If I make a decision to change and listen for my own insights into why I overeat, I have a good chance of changing. If I allow a hypnotherapist to take responsibility for my transformation (implicit in the phrase 'I can make you …') or I pay a coach a significant amount to follow a weight loss programme, then there will always be a part of me that has not decided to take 100 per cent responsibility for my own self-transformation.

Very few people if any discuss the failure rate in the weight loss process. Diet programmes will not do this because if they did, they would put themselves out of business immediately! Most people succeed on diets until they do not. They regain most of the weight, plus interest.

However, if you are lucky enough to have stumbled upon a method that has the potential to work just as well as a diet and which also creates a permanent change, then you have found something where failure is not implicit in the system.

To fail to lose weight following a system like this seems to me to be a problem with the self-transformational nature of insight. Having an insight or not can feel like chasing a fly. How do you know when you have had one? Why is it that all these people are going on about it as if it has changed their life and I really can't relate?

How can I appreciate the importance of insight if I have never had one? How do I know if I have? All of these questions are thoughts.

I watched a great interview recently where someone was being asked how they chose a marriage or a business partner, and they just kept repeating: 'When you know, you know.'

We have all had moments like this in life where we feel that the stars have aligned or we just know that something is right or wrong. This person was describing insight. You have insight when you are able to see something (or hear something) that you know to be true but that you have not seen before. This is usually because you have been approaching the subject with too much thought.

The problem of weight loss has so much thinking involved. Most people who have engaged in it have a head full of contradictory opinions and advice.

It's not surprising that they are unused to listening to themselves from a place of pure wisdom and insight.

So quiet your mind and open yourself to your new thinking. Neither I nor anyone else has the combination to your personal mind lock.

But you do. And that's the point.

Have you ever experienced this form of self-transformation? Are you open to experiencing it now?

FAT THINKING

How hungry am I? Very hungry!

When I see someone who is noticeably overweight or obese, I don't focus on the way they look but rather what they are thinking.

Because I know that what I have termed 'thin thinking' is the way to maintain an appropriate weight; it seems obvious that 'fat thinking' is the nature of the problem.

If we accept the premise that our bodies have a perfect system to keep us slim and healthy, as our thin friends and relatives who never focus on food, then thinking must be getting in the way of us listening to that system.

Having a busy mind, being permanently distracted, or putting too much on our thinking and believing it to be true are all ways in which we can sabotage ourselves.

In the modern world, living from one sugar rush to another leads us to mistake sugar crashes for real hunger, so we end up grazing during the day and eating double or triple the number of meals that our bodies need.

Falling victim to the 'sugar trance' by mistaking processed food for real food is another potential pitfall. Falling victim to advertising and product placement can lead us into habitual consumption of junk food.

Not learning to cook and not equipping our kitchens with appropriate utensils can lead us to air fry or microwave everything that we eat, which therefore leads us to favour processed and ready-to-cook meals.

Letting ourselves decide how much to put on our plates based on how hungry we think we are can lead to chronic overeating—as opposed to putting a little on our plates and discovering how hungry our bodies are and listening to them tell us when we are full.

Overordering take-out food can lead us to empty all the containers that arrive and keep grazing, long after we have eaten our full.

Keeping ourselves distracted whilst eating by watching screens can lead to overeating and eating quickly without chewing a mouthful.

Eating standing up as opposed to sitting with cutlery can lead us to focus on our busy minds, as opposed to what we are eating.

Habitually eating things that do not taste good to us and not chewing our food or allowing our taste buds to savour the flavour of what we are consuming, will lead us to overeat poor quality or bland and tasteless food.

Eating for reasons other than actual hunger—overthinking about food, addictive behaviour, or eating as a result of boredom or loneliness, will lead to overindulging.

As you can see from the above list, the common factor is allowing thinking to get between us and the food we are consuming and between our bodies' natural health and wisdom, which keeps us at our ideal shape.

Do you ever notice your busy mind? Do you catch yourself thinking whilst you eat?

GROUNDING

Where is your experience coming from?
— MICHAEL NEIL

Whenever I feel overwhelmed—in a busy shopping centre, for example—I stop and ask myself this basic question, and my mind immediately slows down.

Grounding is a process that can be described in many ways, but it is used in the world of three-principles coaching to describe the feeling of mental clarity that you achieve when you understand the correct answer to the question above.

Most people will answer this question as if their experience was coming from outside them—'These crowds are making me nervous,' for example. In reality we are creating our experience of reality moment by moment via thought. We are living in the feeling of our thinking and not the feeling of the world.

With this information we can see that we are never, nor can we ever be, the victims of our experiences or of anything else. At least not without our permission.

Ankush Jain, a three-principles coach, runs a workshop where he demonstrates how rare this understanding is. He gives his workshop participants newspapers to read, all of which present reality as if the world really were "outside-in."

Headlines will often describe an event as if it has caused a particular emotion: 'Fury as politician makes statement'; 'Inconvenient event causes anger among motorists.' We know, however, that this description of reality is a misunderstanding of how our experiences work. You can listen to someone speak and feel anger, but it's your thinking about what they have said that creates the emotion, not the other way around. Being triggered—which has become an all-too-popular statement—is itself a misunderstanding.

Being grounded in a correct understanding of reality is a hugely calming and re-assuring feeling. It allows you to manage stress in a highly effective way and to manage your relationships far more effectively because you are far more likely to notice the role of your own thinking in creating your emotional responses.

What I discovered, is that being grounded when I was buying, preparing and eating food, helped to put me in touch with my innate health. Innate health is a concept which is central to an understanding of the Principles. It suggests that there is nothing wrong with us; that our minds play an important role in convincing ourselves otherwise

 ROB SALTER

and that our bodies work perfectly, including in relation to food. We are born with a perfect system for keeping us slim and healthy but we lose touch with it as we age, mainly as a result of excessive thinking.

How would you answer the grounding question right now?

SYD BANKS

*What you are looking for is in the most
hidden place – right under your nose*

– S Y D   B A N K S

In 1973, Sydney Banks, a Scottish welder living in Canada had a profound spiritual experience, which changed his life. He lived for another 36 years, travelling the world and sharing his insights.

Syd essentially understood in a moment of clarity that all of human experience could be expressed by Three Principles: Mind, Thought and Consciousness.

Thought and consciousness work together to give us what we believe is our experience of the world – an outside-in experience, where we feel that the world is acting upon us because we are living in the feeling of our thinking as it moves and changes.

It is only insight – a moment of clarity where we drop 'below' thought and come into contact with Mind – that

   ROB SALTER

allows us to be truly grounded in the truth of life, which is that we are whole, peaceful, loving and healthy.

Syd's mission, as he saw it was to explain this process to as many people as possible, allowing them to experience their true nature.

When I first came across these Principles, I did not 'get it'. Looking back, I now think that this was because I was approaching them with my analytical mind – with thought. It was not surprising that these Three Principles, which seemed so simple, also seemed so difficult to grasp. Was I missing something?

It was not until a number of years later, when I was more stressed than I ever think I had been, that I began to seriously look around at other techniques that I could fall back on, other than the ones that I already knew, which had come up short.

It was at this point that I had my first actual insight, and the Principles, as I had understood them, began to really make sense. I needed to have that visceral experience in order to actually be able to apply my new understanding to the very real problems that I was experiencing in my life at the time.

I was never the same again, as I had found a truth that remains to this day. I can now see where Syd's confidence came from. He knew that all he had to do was to allow people to share the experience that he had, for them to have their own insights.

When you find the key to the lock, you uncover more wisdom than you ever thought possible.

Do the Principles make sense to you right now or are you confused?

THIS UNDERSTANDING CAN CHANGE YOUR LIFE

That's a thought, there's another one!

You may think that you are reading this book in order to lose weight. In reality you are reading this book to get in contact with your personal wisdom.

Your wisdom does not discriminate about the messages that it sends to you. I may have written a book about the messages that my wisdom sent me in relation to controlling my weight. However, I also know that this understanding can produce the most remarkable change in all areas - including pain management, overcoming addiction, managing moods and depression, improving your marriage. The list is virtually endless.

As described in the previous chapter, my first exposure to the Principles was underwhelming, as I responded intellectually to the explanation that I was hearing.

It was only many years later when I was in a highly stressed state and was open to listening to this message again from a more receptive place, that I actually had my first insight. I was listening to a video interview given by Mark Howard when at one point he described a client relating to him how he 'no longer needed to think those thoughts'. I suddenly and spontaneously became aware of myself as a thinking being and had a strong sense that this was not actually my true self.

I still remember driving along and saying to myself: *'that's a thought', that's another thought'* as they drifted across my mind. This insight changed my life. After this I began to keep a journal as more and more insights popped up about all manner of situations that I found myself in.

I realised that I was creating my own experience of life moment by moment via thought and that beneath all that thinking lay my own wisdom, or Mind as it is described in the Principles.

Coming into contact with my own wisdom happened when I was grounded, or not associating with my own thinking. It is sometimes called the Inside Out Revolution because of this realisation that life is coming at us, but from us - that we don't see the world as it is but as we are.

These sayings were no longer cliches or cute quotations for me - they were accurate descriptions of reality. I suddenly understood how to reduce stress, how to find happiness and how to develop my relationships as a result of being

   ROB SALTER

more present to my experience and to my personal interactions.

The insights around weight loss came a lot later, after I had begun to accept that I also had innate health and that I could reclaim it from my habitual thinking around food.

What was your first insight and how did it change you?

HOW INSIGHTS WORK

I have to stop eating my thoughts
The only person who controls
what goes in my mouth is
me and not my diet
Diets must be a misunderstanding
There is no such thing as
good and bad food

In some sense, when you read these actual insights from people that I have spoken to, they appear to simply be common sense. Yet the people who had those insights were transformed by them.

How can this transformation work?

Let's say my action is to over eat at every meal. This happens because I have an emotion of wanting to finish my food, clear my plate, eat a whole portion and maybe ask for seconds.

The emotion comes from a thought - for example - I am very hungry and because I am very hungry I need to eat a lot.

So the process is: thought - emotion - action.

Where does the problem lie then? What is making me fat. My thoughts. That is layer one and that is the layer that The Thin Thinking process deals with.

What is the problem with these thoughts?

They are misunderstandings

What is a misunderstanding? A misunderstanding is based on viewing reality as outside in. So in this case, the thought 'I am hungry and so I need to eat a lot' may not be accurate because when we tune into our stomach and what it is telling us, we may well find once we begin eating, and if we stay in tune with our bodies during this process, our stomach may well send a signal to our brain that we are in fact full and this may come well before we have cleared our plate.

So if we accept that our experience of reality is ultimately inside out - that a true reflection of what our body needs -we can see that often our mind wants to feed us more than our body needs.

Therefore, the insight that *I must stop eating my thoughts* refers to this process of over eating. In fact, on closer inspection it also refers to binge eating and any other addictive behaviour.

'The only person who controls what goes in my mouth is me' is an insight because when we become so confounded by diet thinking' we can convince ourselves that whatever

diet we are following is 'making us' (outside-in) choose one type of food and restricting another. Once we see that this is a misunderstanding and that all this thinking about restriction is simply outside in, we also see how *'all diets are a misunderstanding'* and a corollary of this must be *that 'there is no such thing as good and bad food'* (as diet culture tells us)

So insights transform us because they give us new thought based on a true understanding of reality. It's like being a parcel and being stood the right way up for the first time.

Clear thinking, in line with our wisdom and innate health serves to dispel years of faulty thinking around food and health, which falls away, as we realign with the body that has always been ours to claim.

Once we close all the open tabs in our thinking, we can finally shut down our brains, reboot and restore factory settings.

It's very freeing.

Can you detect the difference between thought and insight? How does each feel different?

 ROB SALTER

WELCOMING INSIGHT INTO YOUR LIFE

Who am I if I don't eat?

If you accept the invitation to allow some new thought into your life, based on a more accurate view of where your experience is coming from, you may find that you have opened a Pandora's Box, as a stream of accompanying 'insights' start to occur to you on a daily basis. My advice is to welcome in this new thought and do not be concerned about having to do anything with them, but rather, allow them to pass naturally and enjoy the process of reframing your experience of eating.

Below are a series of ideas that occurred to me and some which have been shared with me by other people on this same journey. They will often take the form of questions, which come up at meal times:

Am I actually hungry?

Does this feel like genuine hunger or just low blood sugar?

Getting in touch with grehlin and leptin - your body's hunger hormones will recalibrate your body's innate ability to keep you slim

Am I bored?

Sometimes we use food to distract us from unpleasant emotions - these are better experienced and allowed to pass than stuffed down with food

Am I on a sugar roller coaster?

We often snack more after having eaten sugary or processed food

Who am I if I don't eat?

Someone who had just started a diet mentioned this thought to me. She recognised that she had defined herself as 'an overweight person' for years.

Do I like the taste of this?

Once we begin to chew more as opposed to shovelling we may find that we don't like the taste of much of the food that we used to eat.

What taste is this?

When I took the time to research my 5 taste buds (salty, sweet, sour, bitter and unami) I was able to identify the taste combinations that I preferred and try new ones.

Am I tasting my food at all?

My research demonstrated to me that people who ate more slowly and savoured their food were often slimmer

Am I shovelling food?

The opposite was also true! Larger people tended to eat far more quickly

How many times am I chewing?

The difference between shovelling and savouring your food is huge.

Are those people around the table really thinking that about me?

One client of mine had created a whole story about what they assumed her family would say if they saw her change her eating habits. In the end, no one noticed!

Where is my experience coming from in this moment?

This is a great question to ask if you feel that you are distracted and have a busy mind before you sit down to eat.

Is this real food? How many ingredients are there in it? Is it processed? With added sugar?

Whilst I insist in this book that there are no 'good' or 'bad' foods, in terms of dieting - you can lose weight eating virtually anything- there is long term price to pay in terms of our metabolic health from eating a larger proportion of ultra-processed foods.

What would I actually like to eat right now?

As mentioned above, feeling like you have to restrict the foods that you crave can actually be counter-productive)

Do I sit down to eat a meal?

The more likely you are to sit down to eat, the more mindful you are likely to be whilst eating.

I wonder if I can make that dish?

Learning to cook well is a superpower

How would you answer the above questions for yourself? Take your time.

THE TINY WAGON

All diets work - until they don't

Why this process works so much better than a diet.

Imagine for one moment that you have been horribly addicted to drugs or alcohol and good fortune has led to rehab of some kind and you have managed, after years of struggle, to get clean. Then life gets in the way and you find yourself having relapsed and feeling horrible about yourself.

You have 'fallen off the wagon' as the saying goes and the thought of going back to your sober life may seem overwhelming. This is because of the sheer amount of work and soul searching that you had to go through to get to sobriety; the number of people involved in supporting you on your journey. Surely part of the guilt would be to do with how much you have let everyone down.

Something similar happens when we 'fail' on a diet. Because the food that we have been restricting, suddenly seems incredibly appealing, we tend to over eat and that is how dieters who fail often wind up regaining all of the weight that they had lost with interest.

We 'fall off the wagon' as is were and similarly to the experience of an addict, it seems virtually impossible to get back on because we have broken our own rules about what it is that we are restricting. Once the horse has bolted as it were, it seems impossible to return it to the stable.

When I was eating mindfully, I was not restricting any type of food at all. I was simply attending carefully to the process of eating. There were times however, when 'life got in the way' as it often does and I found myself gaining more pounds than I would like. Exactly as in the case with diets, I was unaware that this was happening until I saw my reflection one day and knew that I needed to 'do something'.

It was at precisely this point that I decided to return to becoming mindful about my eating. It felt more like a process of re-calibration than anything else. There certainly was no restriction involved.

I called this process 'getting back on the tiny wagon' because the effort involved seemed minimal. I had not put myself back on a diet, I had not let anyone down and the effort required to attend to my eating, as I had done in the initial weight loss phase of my programme was minimal.

Looking back on how I used to behave - the diet cycle felt like riding a roller coaster. There was nothing calm or measured or indeed mindful about counting calories, or points, or in restricting certain foods. Diets only ever felt temporary to me. However, I had no idea that there was an alternative to restricting food groups or spending countless hours in the gym.

When I explained the Thin Thinking process to one of my clients, I described it this way:

> *Imagine that you are using a calorie counting app - you work out how many calories per day you will allow yourself and you track everything so that at the end of the week you create a calorie deficit. Now imagine that your body can do this for you, without the need of any electronic device. By getting in touch with your ghrelin and leptin signals, you are effectively doing the same thing: you are losing weight via a calorie deficit because you are eating only what your body needs as opposed to what your mind wants to feed you.*

Getting back on the tiny wagon therefore, is simply a matter of attending to your body's natural system for keeping you at your ideal weight.

Have you ever fallen off the wagon? How hard was it to get back on?

DON'T SET GOALS — CREATE HABITS

*It is only a short hop, skip and
jump back onto the tiny wagon*

It feels, looking at the current marketplace of ideas, that habits are most definitely in. It seems like most people have now moved on from goal setting and understood that small, repeatable actions are far more likely to lead to sustainable results in the long term.

I would tend to agree with this sentiment although, in my view, as I have pointed out elsewhere in the book, action is often preceded by emotion and then thought. For me therefore, the correct thinking habits are the key to creating permanent behaviour change.

As I have also demonstrated, when small changes in thought, followed by action are made on a regular basis, results tend to follow an exponential curve and create dramatic changes over time.

The problem with goals therefore is that they tend to specify a time scale, they tend to involve the take up of diets and exercise routines, which simply create their own inherent inertia which undermines all the effort, reverses it and more often than not leads you to a worse position than when you created the goal.

Goals also are unrealistic about failure, self-sabotage and lack of consistency - all things which can be easily overcome using this system because it is only a short hop, skip and jump back on to the tiny wagon.

Most goals tend not to conform to reality and are over ambitious. When I wrote this book for example, I committed to a page a day and for me, this is something that is very do-able. I did not set a time limit or even a specific number of words. I simply created a writing habit that would fit into my existing schedule and lifestyle and would be easy to maintain. It then became motivating to see how far I had come in the first month for example.

When I changed my body, the habit that I took on was to chew my food and to eat when I was hungry and stop when I was full. I found that the one made the other easier. The slower I ate, the more likely I was to notice the signals that my stomach was giving me to either eat or stop eating.

What amazes me then is the regularity with which I see people in the weight loss space talking about goals - food goals, exercise goals and I hear the word 'journey' more often than I care to. It feels as if the combined knowledge of the rest of society has not filtered down to the weight loss world.

I also feel that goal setting puts a lot of people off, who may otherwise take up a micro habit like chewing their food. The idea of chewing what you eat, buying special food, joining a gym, buying workout clothes and so on, is more than many people want to commit to. On the other hand, explain to people that small habits like chewing or walking which can be built into their existing routines without any difficulty can be all that is needed and they will be far more likely to try something new for a period of time, until it has become habitual.

I really wish that this book could be simplified into something as simple as chewing and walking. Or even just chewing because in reality, that is the difference that makes the difference. When I discovered this same truth as part of a self-hypnosis programme, I lost weight quite dramatically and quickly.

I now see a chewing habit is really not something that can be sustained on its own. It does actually need to become part of an insight into the nature of food and eating and what it means to you. This could be a much shorter book, were it really that simple.

Have you ever created a new habit? Did you find it easy to keep to?

INTERNAL V EXTERNAL CALIBRATION

*Does your weight tend
to 'fluctuate, Sir?'*

One popular way to measure your goals is to weigh yourself. However, I had an experience with a particular diet group, which convinced me that regular weighing was not the best idea for me.

I remember the horrible feeling accompanying the weigh in each week. It made me feel so negative about myself when the organisers would fill in my card and I could escape my one or two-pound gain.

The point is that it connected weight loss in my mind with public humiliation. As a result, I did not want to share my weight, nor did I not want anyone else to see what I weighed. Because I had not bought into the diet group's system of points, I was not using it well and on no level did I feel that this system was helping me to lose weight. On the contrary,

I did not find the meetings useful and ultimately I dropped out of the programme and did not return.

There is another major problem with weighing myself which I feel needs to be addressed. I have used scales which have given me widely different readings - literally a 16-pound difference between some scales. As such it is easy to feel that you are making progress, only to be blindsided by a reading that that is wildly higher than elsewhere.

In pure 3P terms, we tend to put way more on to our thinking about the scales measurement than is necessary and that fact that it is virtually impossible to correctly calibrate weighing scales at home.

I tend to associate looking at my 'numbers' with extreme emotions - either elation or depression and this can lead me to extreme behaviour, a desire to restrict food or to over exercise.

When I remember the following it tends to help me relax:

My weight often fluctuates. I can guarantee that I will gain the most weight after a failed diet. I do not want to set goals for myself but rather build routines that feel natural. I want to focus on building habits and routines which support me and I want to eat what I like. Ultimately, I want food to be my friend and not my enemy. I want to build a lifestyle that is sustainable and build regular exercise into that lifestyle and not have to become a gym member, without wanting to. My personal calibration should include photos of me, how

I look in the mirror, how I fit into clothes and what others say about me.

When I follow the rules above and use what I refer to as internal calibration as opposed to the blunt instrument of external calibration, I am more likely to stay happy, emotionally balanced and positive.

Do you have weighing scales? What is your relationship with them?

SEEING THE ROLE OF THOUGHT IN MY OVERWEIGHT

Where we live in a 'sugar trance' ... we consume food which immediately makes us hungry

I began to see that my mind and body were not separate, that my body did not have a mind of its own - on the contrary - it had my mind.

I had a number of insights relating to the role of thought in my body shape and the first was to do with seeing the world as if I were creating my own experience of it moment by moment via thought.

Ironically this is not an insight that you can really 'think your way into'. Like all insight, it comes as a flash of inspiration or knowing. To see me creating my experience of reality, inside out as it were, allowed me to see the inside out nature of everything else that was true about my experience and ultimately to understand that when I perceived the world as 'outside-in', I was fundamentally misunderstanding life.

    ROB SALTER

An example of this would be relationships. I would often ignore the role of my own thinking in my more 'difficult' relationships. Once I began to see that not everyone shared my opinion of certain people and that others may interpret their behaviour in the opposite way to me, I began to see that thought was playing a role in my ability or otherwise to get on with them.

These insights just confirmed the inside out nature of reality to me.

One day I had an insight which shook me. I suddenly could see that every diet I had been on had been a misunderstanding because they were all 'outside-in' - they all were based on the premise that restricting one type of food or adding in one type of exercise was going to change me permanently. I immediately saw why all of these diets had failed - only a change from the inside was going to work long term and this insight allowed me to develop the Thin Thinking principles.

When it came to devising phase two of the principles, I could see that to an extent, I was trying to pursue an outside -in approach by limiting sugar and carbs.

However, on reflection I could see that in reality, all I was doing was to ensure that my innate health -in this case my hunger and fullness response -was actually being disrupted. Any time you restrict a food group, you are overriding the perfect system already in place.

If you operate on a level playing field, you can win the game of health by eating sensibly and reconnecting to your body's innate wisdom in relation to eating what it needs. Where we live in what I term a 'sugar trance' (an outside-in misunderstanding using coloured packaging and marketing to make non-food look edible) we consume food which immediately makes us hungry but in an artificial way, by spiking our blood sugar, so that it crashes soon after each meal.

Ultimately, I simply adopted the tiny wagon approach to carbs and sugar because sometimes, you want to eat complex carbs and sugar and I always let myself do this and simply course correct in my next meal. Most Mediterranean societies operate on this system.

Can you see how insight works in relation to your innate health?

How would your relationships be different if you could drop your incessant thinking?

WHY YOU 'EAT YOUR THOUGHTS' — THE BINGERS

*My desire for the drugs disappeared
as soon as they were in my
hand. I got back to my cell and I
knew that I was an ex-addict*

I once heard a talk from an ex-prisoner, who I will call Charlie, who was describing how learning about the Principles, helped them to overcome an addiction. This person was an excellent raconteur and his gripping story began in the grip of their addiction.

Charlie realised that ultimately, it was the thought of the addictive substance that had them hooked as opposed to the actual substance itself. The incident occurred when they had just spent money on something that they ultimately did not even use.

Like most people who experience a spontaneous insight after coming into contact with the Principles, this person knew that their addiction was over. They came off the substance and began to rebuilding their life, following their own insights.

Mary (not her real name) sat in front of me and described a talk that she has listened to from a 3P practitioner. She was 40 lbs overweight and a binge-eater, bipolar and depressed. Mary cannot pinpoint what it was exactly that changed in her, except for the fact that she had a life altering insight: *'I have to stop eating my thoughts'*.

Mary is sober, sane and 40 lbs lighter.

My insight around my own weight began with one insight and then led to many more. They come like a waterfall and it can be hard to keep up.

It seems that as humans, we were born perfect and have the innate ability to spontaneously heal, whenever we are reminded of who we once were.

When someone takes the time to explain how reality actually works, we spontaneously understand that we have in many ways been complicit in creating a selection of destructive thoughts which have manifested into destructive behaviours.

In a world that wants us to believe that we can ever be victims of anything outside of ourselves, It can seem like we are trapped and that no change is possible.

It always is.

Are you addicted to anything? Can you see the role of thought in your addictive behaviour?

     ROB SALTER

SAVOURING AND YOUR TASTE BUDS

*There I was in this random kebab
shop, groaning with pleasure at the
sheer deliciousness of this meat!*

So far I have spoken in detail about the insights that allowed me to connect with my body's natural system for keeping me slim or my innate health. However, it did not start this way. In fact, I began by using a rather 'outside-in' approach.

I will never forget the day when my friend advised me to count my chews and to try to get to thirty. It felt rather bizarre but the experience of doing so was a visceral one. We happened to be in one of the worst Italian restaurants that I have been to. Of course I did not fully appreciate this fact until I actually started to chew and taste their food.

Prior to this day, we would frequent this restaurant because it is conveniently located and be so busy talking and catching up that I genuinely did not taste any of the food.

Suffice to say that when the waiter asked if I wanted to take home the half a pizza that I had left, I felt very certain that I did not.

As a result of this slowing down and becoming more mindful about eating, I began to rediscover not only my mouth as a centre of digestion but also my taste buds. The corollary of this was that I began to buy food and ingredients based on their taste, as opposed to anything else.

I thought about dishes that I would like to prepare based on their taste and shopped accordingly. When I sat down to eat a meal, I would savour its taste and focus on that, as opposed to the ubiquitous podcast or You Tube video that I would have playing whenever I ate a meal previously.

I cannot stress enough, how this simple but powerfully subtle change, allowed me to shed as much weight as I wanted. At the same time, I began to discover the taste combinations that I preferred and rediscovered my love of certain foods.

Hence the episode mentioned in the brief quote above. I found myself experiencing literal aftershocks of pleasure after a particularly tasty kebab that I ate recently. My Unami taste buds are obviously very powerful sensory receptors and it took a good fifteen minutes for the pleasure to die down after finishing this meal.

One of the experiments that I conducted early on in my research was to observe thin and obese people eating in order to discover if there was a connection with their speed of eating. As I had expected, the thinnest people eat the slowest and the most obese tend to shovel their food. It's not simple process, moving from one body shape to another but the knowledge about the connection to chewing speed can help tremendously in starting a sustainable weight loss process.

Do you shovel or do you savour your food? How difficult do you think it would be to move from one to the other?

POLARITIES

*I am really struggling to lose weight
now I am vegan. It was much easier
before on the Keto diet because
we had all that protein in the
meat but I have changed now*

I have been in the same position as Martha. I also lost weight on a Keto diet. I made a lot of my early content about food from the position of not knowing how to deal with what I called the 'Diet Trap'.

What I meant was that I knew that Keto was unsustainable for me. In fact, I knew that all diets were unsustainable for me. I just did not know that there was any alternative.

I was secretly just waiting for the day when the food that I had been restricting 'took me over' and I ended up at the bottom of a packet of crisps (or three).

It really felt like the food was just waiting to ambush me - that the will power I had been using would finally dry up and I would no longer want to eat just protein and some 'fake' carbs and my cravings for croissants and sourdough would suddenly overwhelm me.

But that sense of impending dread felt so scary and the thought of undoing all the good work that I had done on my diet seemed like such a waste. I could not believe that history was going to repeat itself and I was going to find myself overweight and miserable again, after failing on the same diet that had worked for me over ten years ago.

I waited for what seemed like the inevitable to happen and sure enough - it did. Not only after keto but also after a second calorie tracking diet as well.

Yes, I had ended up fatter than before I started the diet, once again. It felt like being in a car crash in slow motion - you know exactly what is going to happen, but you are powerless to stop it. I felt miserable and ashamed.

When I look back on that period now, a number of things occur to me:

-What would have happened, if instead of going on diets, I just continued to eat normally? I would be in the same place but would have saved myself an awful lot of pain and disappointment?

-Why is it that as soon as we restrict any food group, we automatically begin to crave it and that craving leads us to break the diet?

-How have we got to a point in society, where we have decided that entire food groups must be 'banned'? All animal foods? All carbohydrates? Really? This point is not a criticism of any way of eating but simply an observation that the thought process behind choosing to be a vegan or a carnivore for example is basically the same.

I kept coming back to that little boy who ate everything that he was given, who climbed tress and played football in the park.

He had precisely zero thinking about food. The idea of not eating one type of food, for any reason at all, would have seemed totally weird to him.

Yet as he grew up and began to take on the way that the world has begun to think about food: as if we could add or take one type of food away (or add one type of exercise in) and change our body shape forever.

Had it made him either happier or slimmer?

It did not seem to me that it had.

Quite the opposite.

Have you tried dieting before? What were your experiences?

PLUS-SIZE

*He told me that he was trying hard
to find me physically attractive by
ignoring my plus size shape and
focusing on my personality. I told him
that you should never have to force
yourself to find someone attractive*

I was walking along the street with Judy. She was telling me about the runs that she had been going on after work and it was at that point that she tuned to me and said: *You should get in the gym, Rob.*

When she broke up with me and began dating my friend, he confided in me that my weight was a big factor in Judy deciding to no longer date me.

Similarly, I have heard people comment that once they have lost weight, people do seem to treat them differently. Women for example, who have never been approached by men, suddenly get approached and struggle to cope with the new attention.

It seems that we are programmed to judge others and confer value on them or otherwise, based on their physical shape. We have a lot of thinking about other people's body shape in particular and what it might mean.

This is one reason, I believe why the movement to accept people whatever they look like, has taken hold.

It seems completely unfair, prejudiced even, to make a judgement on someone's worth as a human being, based on their size.

Why could Judy not see past my overweight and continue to date me, for example? Why did she think that it was okay to comment negatively on it?

If I think back and ask myself why I had gained weight at that point, I can think of numerous reasons, mainly to do with extra stress, which had not put me in a good place mentally and emotionally.

I had been comfort eating for a while. My father had become ill and my family were making many hospital visits.

The thinking that got me to the size that I was at was not happy. Looking back, I did not fundamentally disagree with what Judy was saying.

Because I had been used to being slim and fit myself, this new more sedentary and stressed Rob was new to me and was an unwelcome visitor.

When I look back now, however insulting it seemed at the time, Judy was only saying out loud, what I probably felt about myself.

Were we both misunderstanding reality? Is it always wrong to judge others based on superficial criteria?

It's a hard thing to admit but that was not the thinking that helped me to lose the weight and for me to become too attached to it and to make it my personality, in sheer reaction to a negative comment was just not something that had ever occurred to me.

When I put too much on any thought I have about my size - when I believe everything that I think, I get myself into trouble. When I observe my thinking, particularly if there are strong feelings attached to it, I become suspicious.

I live in the feeling of my thinking and my thinking changes as do my feelings.

My thinking did change about weight and as a result, I lost a lot that sadness around my waist.

People did respond to me differently and to an extent, I accepted that my new size reflected my new thinking.

If I start from the position that I have innate health and that my body already knows how to keep me slim then any overweight I have is a result of me 'eating my thoughts' to a degree.

Perhaps that is what people are 'seeing'?

Perhaps we are not so much objectivising others bodies, than responding to their 'plus size' thinking about themselves?

What is your thinking around your own body image?

 ROB SALTER

I AM A TUMOUR CARRIER

Read that phrase again. Sounds wrong doesn't it?

From the age of 55 I contracted diabetes and bladder cancer. I thought of them as my leaving gift from my teaching career. I have a sense of black humour. What can I tell you?

When my tumour was found, it was removed mercifully quickly and I still have yearly scans to make sure that it does not return. When a blood test showed that my blood glucose was elevated I was told that I was a diabetic and was given a leaflet called 'living with diabetes'. There was no talk of a cure, or remission or reversal. It was all about stepping on the merry go round of nurses, medications, eye tests, etc. It felt like there was a special club, just waiting for me to join, with a badge and a t-shirt with 'I am a diabetic' printed on it.

I do, of course, understand the difference between the two diagnoses.

I know that having a cancerous tumour in your body has little if anything to do with my lifestyle choices. I do also understand that the thinking about food that got me my diabetes diagnosis is very common and is, theoretically at least, hard to change. I say 'the thinking that got me here' because it really is thinking that got me to eat emotionally and to routinely choose ultra-processed, convenience food over whole food.

It was thinking about stressful situations that got me to raise my cortisol levels which in turn chronically raised my blood glucose levels. It was my thinking about exercise that kept me out of the gym, kept me in my car and made me stop at every service station on the journey to and from work, for snacks. It was my thinking that convinced me that momentarily spiking my blood sugar was going to somehow, magically 'make me feel better'.

So presumably, it would be my thinking that got me out of this 'diagnosis' and would allow me to hand back the t-shirt and the leaflets, despite the fact that the UK health service seemed keen to welcome me into the diabetic's club, as did the Diabetic Facebook groups.

What I can say is that this new thinking, to the extent that I embraced it, got me scared. It got me to try and fail on two diets and to end up fatter than I had been. Far from helping me, it led me back into a diet culture that had failed me in the past. The only difference this time, is that the level of fear was greater. I felt like I could not afford to fail, having listened to the horror stories about people suffering with untreated diabetes for too long. We've all heard and been scared by the horror stories.

It was only when I began to approach the issue of the thinking itself, my fat thinking as I like to call it, that I was able to lose a lot of the weight and keep it off. It was only when I began to approach my thinking about my body and how I was not using it as intended, that I began to walk, cycle, skip and run again.

The thinking I had around diabetes and what it meant I could or could not eat turned out to be supremely unhelpful. Mainly because, as outlined elsewhere in this book, it simply became a list of 'banned' foods that I inevitably began to crave; far more than if I had never tried banning them in the first place.

Ultimately, diabetes describes a range of numbers on a blood test. Like my scale weight, those numbers fluctuate, meaning that I could be normal on a Friday but pre-diabetic on a Wednesday. What really matters is the way that I approach my thinking about these readings and about my health in general.

Once I began to detach from the over thinking around health and disease that our culture insists on, I had the mental bandwidth to attend to my moment by moment experience of my body and listen to the wisdom it was sharing with me.

That is when I began to recover.

Have you been diagnosed as diabetic? What has your experience been?

'BAD' FOOD

My first girlfriend's mum used to eat fresh white bread with butter. I have not allowed myself to eat that for years because I was convinced it was bad for me. I had some yesterday and it was amazing!

Can food ever actually be 'bad'?

When I used to drive to work and have a sausage and egg Mc Muffin every morning for breakfast, was I being a bad person? Or was I simply attaching the idea of a 'treat' for having to wake up at 6.30am and drive for 35 minutes on the A406 to get to work? When I would regularly eat take-aways because I was too tired to cook, was I also being 'bad' by eating 'bad' food.

When I first started working with clients, I got them to re-acquaint themselves with their taste buds. To experiment with bitter, salty and unami foods. To see which combinations they preferred and to let their shopping habits be guided by their taste buds.

Food can be 'whole' or 'ultra-processed' and we cannot always help eating convenience or take away foods. My contention is that this is unavoidable but that if we are guided by our taste buds, then we will gravitate away from sugar laden, bland tasting products, towards whole and healthy choices -just based on taste alone.

My mum would never want to take us to restaurants because as she used to say: 'I could cook better at home'. The better I got as a cook, the less I ate out as well.

When I was buying and eating 'junk' I was not chewing or savouring what I ate - I was eating my thinking and my emotions. I was tired, frustrated and unhappy and I used food as a reward. For me the answer was to change the circumstances of my life and then retrying to eating with a blank slate. It was not 'bad' food because food is just food.

The idea that food can ever actually be 'bad' is just that - an idea. It's a thought. We may attach emotions to that thought, which connect eating 'bad' food with being 'naughty' or even a 'bad person'. Once again, if we do that, we are putting way too much on our thinking, rather than just allowing ourselves the necessary slack to exist in the modern world of factory farming and multinational food companies.

Living and working in France taught me a lesson that I can never forget: that it matters far more how you eat than what you eat. That you can eat a diet high in fat, in meat, in bread and pastries and still stay slim. That if you focus on the rituals of meal times and savour your food and take time over eating it then your body can make far better use of whatever you are feeding it.

The corollary of this idea is that you want to be eating food that is worth sitting down for! Fast food restaurants have Drive Thru's for a reason. Like a petrol station you are refuelling, often eating in your car.

If anything, there may be bad eating habits -as promoted by the 'fast food culture' that we live in - as opposed to 'bad' food as such.

Perhaps what I really learned in France was how to value the whole process of shopping, cooking and eating, rather than farming out responsibility for all of it to fast food companies.

Now I basically eat what I want. I no longer believe in either 'good' or 'bad' food because I know that I can mitigate for the occasional take away during the rest of the week.

I believe that I can now maintain my shape because I have learned to let my body tell me what I need rather than let my mind over feed me.

If I do eat take away. I still tend not to over eat.

And that is the key.

Do you have fixed ideas about what 'good' or 'bad' food would be?

 ROB SALTER

DROWNING IN NOISE

*When I listen to you, it helps
you to listen to yourself*

Everybody knows how to lose weight. If you ask ten people, they will all say versions of the same thing. My contention is that this is because they are all simply repeating what they have heard out in the world. There is an orthodoxy about weight loss which kind of drowns out any other thinking. It seems like 'common knowledge'

The one thing that all the advice has in common is simply that it is based on a model of the world and an understanding of where our experience is coming from that is 'outside-in'.

My contention is that this is a misunderstanding of how reality actually works, which is 'inside out'.

My very first insight was about precisely this - every piece of advice I have heard is based on adding in or restricting food groups or adding in various forms of exercise. My contention is that, we are already perfect and have innate health. Our bodies have a built in system for keeping us slim.

It's not something that is accessible by thought, by diet, by exercise. It's something that we are either in touch with or not. I know this because there are many people that I know (and I am sure that you know as well), who are 'naturally' slim and who eat what they want.

My contention is that these people, mostly without realising it, are in touch with their innate health - with their body's natural system for keeping us slim. In order to lose weight permanently then, we need to tap into that innate health too.

When I work with clients, I listen to them deeply and I ask them to articulate their particular problem as they see it. This is because I want to give them the time and space, within a coaching session, for their thinking to calm down and for them to actually listen to themselves - and to listen from a deeper place. This deeper listening will often result in an insight - a sight from within.

Once they are 'connected up' as it were, to this new and strange paradigm, they are then open to hearing more about their own innate health. At this point then, the innate ability that we all have to listen to the signals that our stomach is giving us will allow people to eat in a more 'natural' way.

They will begin to see that what they eat is far less important than how they eat. The more time they spend and attention they put on the process of eating, the more they will get in

 ROB SALTER

touch with what their bodies actually need as opposed to what their mind wants to feed them.

As a result of this new understanding, the old outside in paradigm can fall away. It's not an easy thing to drown out the noise, which our brains tend to record over time and file under 'facts'. It takes time and patience to move away from the various traps that this paradigm sets for us.

Here is Rabbi Johnathan Sacks on this idea: '*live simply. Don't eat more than you need. Don't drink more than you need. Don't spend more than you need. Never buy something simply to impress others – they may say they're impressed but they aren't. Isn't it strange that in the 21st-century people spend fortunes on diets, exercise, machines, and personal trainers to lose the weight, they would not of put on if they stopped eating when they were satisfied?*' 'Investing Time' 2012 - United Synagogue Publications.

Do you stop eating when you are full? Do you ever leave food on your plate?

MY BIRTH RIGHT

No pain - no gain

I sat in the cafe and watched a short, middle aged and rather dumpy woman book a personal training session with the toned, muscular PT at the laptop. Clearly this guy was the exercise alpha dog of the local area.

So far, so normal.

Except after leaving the cafe, I had an insight. *'Good health and fitness do not belong to that guy. They belong to everyone'.* To be honest, at that point, I did not exactly know what I meant by that insight: when they come, insights are often not 'whole'. Over the next days, however, I began to realise that what I had witnessed in that cafe was thought: his thoughts about health and fitness and hers.

Essentially they both were agreeing that he 'had it' and she 'did not'. The woman looked like the average busy, stressed but wealthy middle class mum, who could afford a personal trainer.

My insight was that it was impossible to 'not have' your birthright. It belongs to you and is waiting for you to claim. Personal training is an outside in approach and misses the point whilst reinforcing the misunderstanding that you don't have what you already do.

The journey to claiming it is an internal one. Your version of health and fitness may never involve gym wear. Many heathy, fit and long living people, many of whom live in the so called Blue Zones, have never seen a gym.

Were they to meet someone with that classic V body shape, built in the weights room of a gym, they would be bemused at why anyone would choose to look like this.

Innate health looks different for everyone. All children look different but are essentially healthy and fit. They live in tune with their bodies and with the world around them.

Once, as adults we accumulate years upon years of extraneous thought about how we should look and how we should 'discipline' ourselves to remain healthy and fit, we lose touch with our innate health. Then we succumb to the messages that society sends us about what is appropriate to eat and what is 'quick and easy'.

We bulk up and we try to shed. Balance and equilibrium are long gone. We shovel rather than eat - glued to our distraction machines while we do so. We look at our expanding waistlines with bemusement and then take out our latest gym membership.

The world we live in leads us to surrender our innate health to others. To the food manufacturers, the gyms and personal trainers who then commoditise and sell our own 'heath' back to us at a premium price.

The process by which we can reclaim our innate health necessitates slowing down. It requires us to step off of the hamster wheel of business and productivity for a moment and see the wood for the trees.

It points us back to our childhood, to a world without any extraneous thought about either food or exercise. It requires us to be free.

So what does innate health look and feel like?

I remember making one very powerful distinction early on in my weight loss journey: *I am not exercising in order to lose weight. I am exercising because I have lost weight.*

There is major difference between the two frames of mind. The first frame is what we see online when people begin to 'Glow Up'. The problem as far as I see it, is that these people are basically swapping one extreme for another. They go from obesity to being shredded. There does not seem to be any moderation in their behaviour.

When I began to exercise, the first thing that I did was to park my car and walk. I invested in walking shoes and made walking a part of my daily experience. I loved it. My body loved it. Over time, as I slimmed down I did spend a little time in the gym but it was always as an adjunct to what I

　　　　　　　ROB SALTER

was already doing in the kitchen and at the dining table. I was mindful of the maxim that you can never outrun a bad diet and I did not try.

There is one (rather brutal) test that I developed recently to determine who is using their body as intended. I call it the Yes/No test. Sit in a large car park one day and then the next day sit in a town centre, preferably one that can only be reached by public transport or walking. Then look at the people walking by and ask yourself if they are physically proportional at the 'right' body weight for their height. Make a fairly superficial assessment by saying 'Yes' or 'No' -to yourself (!)- and see how your assessment differs where people access the environment in their cars. I will let you draw your own conclusions.

Do you have a gym membership? How do you feel about exercise?

DISEASE PROMOTING CULTURES

Since arriving in Europe. I have been walking everywhere and eating food that does not kill me. I've literally deflated. I hate America

I arrived in LA as a student and quickly discovered that I was the only person in the city without a car. I ended up cycling around the city because I had not qualified as a driver. I clearly remember the intense heat - there was a heatwave that year and the strange looks that I would get from other drivers.

I still left America ten pounds heavier.

Twenty years later, I was wandering around Orvieto in Tuscany and came upon the evening 'passagiata'. The whole town seemed to be out walking after dinner, buying gelato, smoking cigars and chatting. Similar to my experience in France, I seemed to do little but eat amazing food and still lost weight as a result of simply participating in European culture.

When I decided to change my life, my first realisation was that I did not own a pair of walking shoes. I was so used to hopping in and out of my car - which I overused tremendously - that I had rarely walked for more than 20 minutes at a time.

I found that my shoes and my Apple Watch are the two best investments that I have made in my health. If I go for a run or visit the gym nowadays it's not because I want to exercise in order to lose weight, I exercise because I've *already* lost weight.

When I gave my car away, I moved to a new city with great public transport. Once back in London, I resisted the temptation to buy a new car and just decided that it was worth walking that little bit further, in order to get from A to B in a big city.

Modern Industrialised societies are used to commoditising most things. Thus, real food is bastardized, packaged and marketed back to you in a convenient format. Similarly, your health is commoditised and sold back to you as gym wear and memberships, personal trainers and spin classes.

Old people in Orvieto may well live beyond 100 because their city has steep steps. They are used to walking and eat freshly prepared food. The idea of heating a ready meal in a microwave or going to a spin class may make them laugh, or even cry.

When I lost my weight, I did a great deal of research into these cultures and how they cope if they need to lose some pounds. Most of the time, people had simply slipped out the rhythm of life as dictated by their traditional society. All they needed was a re-calibration.

For us in the industrialised West, we need to first understand how our culture is keeping us fat and then how to undo the damage.

Do you consume mainly processed food? Do you cook from fresh ingredients?

THERE ARE TWO VERSIONS OF YOU

*If we want to help people we
have to forget about helping
them; that's the paradox*

-JACK PRANSKY

Jack Pransky is a Three Principles coach who is clear on the limits of coaching anyone using this approach to coaching. When it comes to coaching weight loss clients, I am always mindful of his words.

The version of me that lost my weight initially was not a working man. The version of me that put it back on was. To be precise, that 'second' version of me, once back at work, found it significantly harder not to believe my own thinking. I struggled to not feel a victim of my circumstances. I struggled not to comfort eat and undo all the good work that my previous self, had accomplished.

Despite the fact that 'enlightened me' already knew not to attach too much to my thinking and knew that I was creating my experience of the world, moment by moment via thought, I still indulged my own 'fat thinking' on numerous occasions and found myself inhaling crisps, chocolate and take-aways in order to 'make myself feel better'.

This is why some of my clients did not lose weight. This is also why some people lose a large amount of weight after gaining an insight into an area of their lives that might seem to be totally divorced from their 'presenting problem' of over-weight.

It was my thin thinking, which allowed me to recalibrate my relationship with food. However, had I experienced a major change in my thinking about the work that I do, or in some cases the ability to quit a problematic job, or make a life-changing amount of money, that could have become the lever that I needed to shed my own pounds.

It's not unusual to hear of people who become financially successful and drop 40 lbs without thinking about it. It's the deconstruction of the second, stressed, victimised self that has allowed their true selves to shine through.

As a coach then, to come to this process with only weight loss in mind can be a huge mistake. -If there really are two of me, I need to accept that only one of them may be 'thinking thin'.

Jack Pransky is clear that a coach must listen deeply to their client and work with what the client gives them and not lead them towards the Principles if they are not ready. I can attest to the importance of this when I remember my initial reaction to hearing about 'Mind, Consciousness and 'Thought'. These ideas meant very little to me when I approached them purely as intellectual concepts.

Similarly, when I hear other people describe their own insights or I explain mine to others, I am painfully aware that I may just be exposing myself or others to more 'noise'. Pure insight works on a level of knowing that lies beneath thought. An insight is a spontaneous process that cannot be controlled or directed. It enlightens you in ways that you could not have imagined and which you cannot predict.

However, the power of insight is that whenever it occurs, whatever it illuminates, it may create a ripple effect which can effect profound change in any sphere of life.

That is why insights are worth waiting for.

Do you find it harder to maintain your weight when you are stressed and working?

THERE ARE NO VICTIMS

If I was single, I'd be three stone lighter. My wife is a feeder and she buys all the bad stuff

This quote from an early client of mine sums up everything that comes from our investment in believing that reality is 'outside-in'. When I answer the grounding question from the point of view of someone who is reacting to the outside world and who believes that what happens outside of me can in some way change me, I in some way define myself as a victim.

It's far easier to blame others, the weather, the economy or whatever for our problems than to take responsibility for our own experience and change ourselves. We have to give others permission for them to 'change' us. My client for example would prefer to blame his wife for his behaviour towards him because on some level, it absolves him of responsibility for his own transformation.

When I slip out of the awareness that I am describing in this book, I also sometimes feel like the victim of the 'food environment' that I live in. I can feel a victim of product placement in supermarkets, of the food industry in general, of advertising and marketing and so on. I can feel like the victim of my job, which stresses me and 'makes' me comfort eat. I can feel like the victim of the hours I work and of my long commute to work.

The list is endless. Here is the point. Each sentence above begins with the words 'I can'. The implication is that I always have a choice. I may not always make the 'right' choice for me. However, the alternative is to 'force' myself to restrict a specific food group for a specific amount of time, or to force myself into Lycra for a gruelling work out/punishment session. The result is that, as a result of feeling like a victim I then choose to victimise myself as a 'logical' response to weight gain.

Humans are imperfect creatures and if we do not work in a way which complements our basic nature, we rebel and self-sabotage. Punishing ourselves for doing this misses the point completely. The point lies in how we see reality as a whole, in how we answer the grounding question for ourselves. If innate health is our birthright and if our bodies have a perfect system for keeping us slim, then surely all we really need to do is to clear our minds long enough to allow that system to work.

My body knows what it needs and when it needs it. It knows when to eat and when to stop eating. It knows which foods make it feel most alive and which make it feel sluggish. My tongue is blessed with taste buds, which point me to the tastes and flavours that I like.

The 'bad stuff' that my client referred to - ultra processed snack food -is something that I also indulge in from time to time. My mind tells me that these foods are often brightly coloured and appealing. Its tells me that they are also laden with sugar and salt, to make me want more. The answer to his question really is that, having something in the house that is not good for me is not the same as me making the choice to eat it.

I am not a victim. I can choose to say yes or no. I can choose to ignore what is there or to allow myself to eat. The actions of others will not ultimately decide the fate of my health because I never be a victim without my permission.

The 'bad' food in the cupboard can stay there. If my family members are feeders, I can eat - until I have had my full.

Is there anything in this chapter that resonates with you? Have you ever felt like you were a victim and had no choice in a particular situation? Can you see how victimhood is a choice? Take your time.

THE IMPORTANCE OF BREAKING BREAD

You always eat well at Carlo's ... But I digress

ADRIANO GALLIANI,
explaining how he persuaded Ancelotti to
sign as a manager for AC Milan Football
Club (and being distracted by the food)

I could not work out why my weight loss clients were not losing weight. Then I read something that knocked me for six. As a society, we have become addicted to a virtual experience of ourselves and of each other.

People remember meals. Not video calls.

The great manager Carlo Ancelotti's first move when attempting to turn around the fortunes of PSG football club was to create a small restaurant, to mimic that of AC Milan where waiters serve the players food and a manager can experiment with seating players next to different team mates, so that they can bond and become a cohesive unit.

The sporting director of AC Milan remembers precisely the food that Carlo served him after they had sealed that piece of business.

I realised that I needed to eat with my clients. This one change did more for my business than anything else. When I was not reaching them was when I was trying to communicate via screens. People need to experience each other in a visceral way - face to face. If they can break bread together, they have already bonded.

Coaching and helping others is ultimately about connecting. You can't really see where a client needs to go next if you are not physically with them. You can't teach people about food if you are not sharing an experience of eating together.

Connecting with your innate health, with the subtle messages that your body is sending you, is a subtle change process. Subtle but profound. Learning to leave some food on your plate and how that communicates meaning to your brain is also a subtle distinction.

I was lost in my business when it was purely online. I was promoting something that no one was looking for, among a sea of people who all believe that they 'know how to lose weight but just can't consistently do what they know'. I was competing in a polarised world full of carnivores, vegans and precious little in between. There were glow up videos, muscled gym addicted personal trainers wanting you to look like a version of them.

After I while I realised that I had to build this, one relationship and one meal at a time. I had to do less coaching and more eating. People could read my book and then decide if their experience with me was worth pursuing.

Do you regularly eat with and cook for others?

FAILURE IS YOUR BEST TEACHER

Try again. Fail again. Fail better
-SAMUEL BECKETT.

I recently had a five week backslide during last March and it was the failure that allowed me to refocus and ultimately massively improve my approach and ultimately my weight loss.

School is not a great teacher in the sense that it stigmatises failure when in fact this is the one thing that is the most useful to us in life, although in school when we receive a cross or a 'bad mark' we are encouraged to believe that this is a reflection on us as individuals.

In reality failure is a wonderful teacher, particularly in weight loss. Failure gives us the opportunity to reflect on what has gone well and what needs to be improved.

For me it allowed me to finally find the missing piece of my jigsaw. It allowed me to have an insight around the concept known as intermittent fasting and finally see how, as a concept, it fits perfectly into the eating system that I had already created for myself and that I present now.

One problem that I encountered on my weight loss journey was the amount of weight that I was able to lose at one time. Initially, I was able to lose ten kilos relatively easily. However, the problem that I encountered, even when I had reached my initial goal was that my blood work still showed that diabetes was present.

Adding in intermittent fasting allowed me to lose as much as fifteen kilos, which is the amount of weight that I needed to lose in order to reverse my diabetes. The extra ten kilos made all the difference and allowed me to set a new set point for my body.

So how does 'fasting' fit into the system that I had already intuited? It actually has everything to do with being present to your own feelings of hunger. In the past, I would eat breakfast, whether I felt actual hunger or not. The only real change in my new version of this system was that I did not eat until around midday or 1pm and I also made sure not to snack after dinner. In fact, I reduced snacking completely, so that I was mainly eating square meals at each meal time and not between meals.

What I realised was that in many respects it was only my thinking which led me to eat before midday and to snack between meals. My body's hunger cues were not telling me to eat before then.

Why have I included a chapter on failure, on backsliding? Because natural weight loss has to also be seen in the context of natural weight gain. This could be as a result of a prolonged period where you simply lose touch with what your body wants and needs and become enmeshed in your own thinking. It can be as a result of Developing a pattern of addictive eating of ultra-processed food. There are an unlimited number of food traps out there - and unlimited opportunities to comfort eat with the hope that that thing outside of yourself will change how you feel.

Learning to see the world the right way up, as our experience being created by us, is going to be a lifelong struggle. Yes, you can circumvent this process with a smart drug, a GLP1 for example, but ultimately the struggle that I outline in this book is the real struggle of life in my view. Fighting the good fight is a lifelong struggle but one that is worth winning.

What have you learned from life's failures?

ENTER THE FAST

*"Fruit does not get digested
in the stomach"*

-HARVEY DIAMOND

In 1985, Harvey and Marilyn Diamond wrote a book which changed my life. Fit for Life allowed me to drop weight and keep it off for many years.

Once I had 'left' the programme, one thing remained for many years after, which helped me to Stay slim and that was to eat 'fruit till noon' as the programme taught me. Fruit is digested in the mouth and small intestine and so you are effectively fasting each day until midday if you follow this system.

If you stop eating after dinner the night before, say around 8pm, then you have fasted for 16 hours without realising it. Once again, I tend to eat fruit if I am hungry, breaking the Fit for Life orthodoxy but allowing me to fast from after dinner onwards.

Now you will occasionally crave some kind of breakfast and when this happens I normally allow myself to eat. By the same token however, if I hold off and do not react to the hunger pang, then I can stay 'not hungry' way past midday. The craving is more often than not a simple sugar dip that can be recognised as such and understood for what it is.

By way of contrast, when I was getting into work at 7am, I would always visit McDonalds for a McMuffin breakfast. Is breakfast really the most important meal of the day or was this simply a marketing ploy to serve the food companies. It certainly added inches to my waistline.

Once again, when I aimed to wait until midday before eating any solid food, the weight seemed to drop off.

The final piece of the jigsaw was the relationship between fasting and food noise. One major lesson to come out of the GLP1 debate was the way that this medication deals with 'food noise' - this is the constant mental chatter around food that we experience when we are over taken by our busy minds.

The strange thing about fasting until noon is the effect that this has on food noise in general. I may 'feel hungry' at around eleven am but if I allow myself to think about other things then I find that I can go without eating until one or two pm without any problem. It turns out that the 'hunger cue' was more like a sugar dip and probably not real hunger at all.

You may think about fasting and worry that you won't be able to do it, but it's important to remember that these are really only thoughts. Once you get into the swing of it, it does not feel difficult at all.

Have you ever tried fasting? How has it worked for you?

WHEN YOU RETURN TO YOUR FACTORY SETTINGS

Everyone is telling me how slim I look

I get it. Really I do. I am supposed to be the expert. I am supposed to have all the answers. I don't.

I am literally eating what I want, when I want. The scales tell me I have gained a few pounds. The scale readings don't mean that much to me. There is no emotional response to this information where there would have been previously.

Everyone is telling me how slim I look. The mirror in the bathroom (and other bathrooms) likes me again. Full length mirrors love me.

I stopped attending to how often I chew months ago. I see myself eating faster again than other people around me. And yet I am still slim. How has this happened? Surely this is against 'the rules' - even mine.

I really only have one explanation and its a pretty flimsy one so bear with me.

I feel that I my body has been returned to its factory settings and is basically behaving as it did before I 'got fat'.

I do notice two major changes:

I don't really snack between meals. I eat if I feel hungry and I don't eat if I don't. I walk a lot and take every opportunity to get closer to 'closing my rings' on my Apple Watch.

Crucially however I now find it quite hard to over eat. Yesterday for example I got a takeaway and I left a fair amount of it. Have a physical memory of the last time I had this food and ate it all and I literally felt like I was going to vomit.

The other week I over ate deliberately for a specific reason and I also felt awful the next day.

If I add all this up I would formulate it this way:

Restoring factory settings means that you become far more in tune with your grehlin and leptin responses. You become far more aware of when you are hungry and when you are full.

Because you are no longer eating your thoughts, eating with your eyes - whatever you want to call it - because your mind is no longer feeding you more than your body needs, your body is actually regulating your weight for you.

Which is what it is meant to do.

I started this way of eating just over a year ago, because I was sick of failing on diets and realised that, as a diabetic, I could not afford to fail.

I calibrated what 'normal' eating looked like and slowed my own eating down considerably. I observed people eating. I researched how other cultures consumed food. I suspected that my body -having innate health - would have a perfect system for keeping me slim, which my busy mind was not listening to.

I now believe that I my hunch was correct and that once the calibration is complete, my body will slip back into its normal state and keep me slim.

Despite not completely understanding, it's a wonderful feeling.

Have you returned to factory settings? Does this feel in any way like a 'new you'?

 ROB SALTER

GLOSSARY

3P: The Three Principles, as articulated by Sydney Banks – Thought, Consciousness and Mind

Insight: A sight from within, a flash of inspiration or knowing where you see reality as it is, beyond thought. In relation to 3P an insight occurs when we see beyond the illusion that Thought and Consciousness create for us.

Outside-in: A misunderstanding of reality that most of us live in. We feel that life is happening to us, that we are victims of other people and circumstances.

Inside-Out: The true nature of our experience. We create our experience of the world via thought and we live in the feeling of our thinking. Insights tend to come to us as experiences of ourselves as thinking beings.

Innate Health: A concept within the 3P world that there is nothing wrong with us, either physically or mentally. We have perfect health, which is our birthright. Most illness and disease is thought created.

<u>Ghrelin</u> – a hormone, secreted by your stomach that tells you that you are hungry

<u>Leptin</u> – a hormone that tells your brain when you have eaten enough.

<u>Unami</u> – it means 'delicious savoury taste' in Japanese and is one of your five taste buds. It detects meat and other savoury flavours.

<u>Sugar Trance</u> – the name I use to describe the glucose roller coaster, where we eat sugar laden food, which does not fill us up, but instead makes us crave more sugar-rich foods.

THIN THINKING COURSE ON TEACHABLE

Have you failed on diets?

Have you given up? Have you accepted your larger body?

Do you have a wardrobe full of clothes you cannot wear?

I'm about to tell you a secret: you can have that body you always wanted. You can eat what you want. You don't need to commit to a lifelong diet

You don't even need drugs to do this

You can become healthier. You can watch as your body becomes athletic. You can glow up for good and never look back.

Don't let anyone tell you it's impossible. Don't let anyone tell you that it's easy.

This is the important part - you won't want to miss this

This system involves a paradigm shift: a mental revolution.

This hack is so simple it can literally be achieved by answering one question

The correct answer will change your life because it will put you in touch with your body's natural blueprint for keeping you slim.

Suddenly your naturally slim friends won't seem so lucky after all. Once you understand this secret that even they don't know about, their lifestyle - the one you have always envied- will be open to you.

And here's the best part:

Once you have the correct answer, not only will you begin to see your body physically transform but you may find discover a ton of other benefits that you had NOT expected

- you will be able to handle stress
- Your relationships will improve
- Your addictions will release their hold over your mind
- You will not be nearly as bothered by the 'food noise' that locked you into obesity.

That is lifetime value!

As you can probably imagine - this all seems too good to be true. No one is looking for this because the food and diet industries want you looking in the opposite direction.

They want you looking at short term fixes, the ones that you know only produce short term results - why? Because then you become a lifetime customer.

How much does this all cost?

The price and the value will amaze you.

That's it. No strings.

What's in this for me?

That's a great question

Basically I am one of the ONLY people on the planet right now who is prepared to take this powerful wisdom and apply it to weight loss. When people begin to create their own success, the financial benefits will appear for me, as the diet industry finally wakes up to the fact that they are losing customers.

For now, my priority is to get this powerful information into the hands of the largest number of people and allow them to roll with it.

Access the course here: https://rob-salter-s-school.teachable.com/p/thin-thinking